Allergy Free Today

For Children and Adults

Aaron Orpelli, DC

Edited by Kayte Deioma

Dedication

I dedicate this to my wife, Eva, and my children—Naomi, David and Sara. You are the lights of my life.

Acknowledgments

Thank you to all of my fellow doctors and colleagues, past and present, here in the United States and around the world, who are working to develop and spread the greatest healing modalities in the world.

Special thanks to the following chiropractors, who have shared their knowledge and enthusiasm with me: Dr. George Goodheart, Dr. Victor Frank, Dr. Scott Walker, Dr. Timothy Francis, Dr. Walter H. Schmitt, and Dr. Devi Nambudripad. Dr. Thurman Fleet's practice and research clarified my practice to identify the weakest system in the body first.

I am also grateful to my staff at Allergy Free Today in Los Angeles, California.

It is with great love and appreciation that I extend the warmest thanks to all of my patients, without whom this book would not have been possible. They helped me become the allergy elimination expert I am today.

Many thanks to Craig Duswalt for giving me the motivation and encouragement to write this book.

Foreword

I am excited to share my personal experience and research, as well as the teachings of great doctors and pioneers who came before me in the specialty of allergy elimination. My goal is to create hope and tools for individuals to be healthy, happy and to experience life to the fullest, and to help parents raise the next generation of optimally healthy kids. By living your lives to your greatest potential, you will become an example of health for the world.

This book will guide you to eliminate your own allergies and help your children heal from any allergies they may have. It will provide methodologies that can start eliminating allergies immediately and put you on a path to becoming allergy free today. I will provide information to guide you in choosing the right doctor to help you eliminate those allergies permanently.

Contents

Chapter 1: The Child

"Failure is success if we learn from it."
--Malcolm Forbes

It was night when my fever spiked and the familiar pain was back. I was exhausted, but could not sleep. It hurt to pee and there was blood in my urine. I was just nine years old. I had been home for just three days after a one-month stay in the hospital. It had started with a skin infection that moved to my kidneys and refused to heal. We thought it was better, but now it was back.

My parents bundled me up and put me in the car for the 30-minute drive back to the hospital. I asked my dad to stop the car on the way because I had to throw up. I was weak and shaky. I could not get comfortable.

At the hospital, the doctor welcomed me and introduced me to the nurse. She took me to change my clothes and led me to my bed. My parents said goodbye and left me there, alone.

The ward was cold and white. The first time I was in this ward, my bed was just a couple beds from the door, almost as close as you could be to the exit. This time, I was by the far wall. The door seemed so far away that I felt no hope of reaching it to get out.

In the morning, I saw other kids getting up out of their beds and playing games or with toys, but the nurse sent me back to bed. She told me what my new routine would be. They wake us up at 5 o'clock in the morning to give us medication, and then we go back to sleep until breakfast at seven. I felt very weak and had no problem falling back to sleep.

Most of the children would eat breakfast at a table. At the beginning, they let me eat at the table too, but later, because my kidney infection did not improve and my blood pressure stayed high, they made me stay in bed to have my meals. I felt isolated and lonely but the doctors were worried that I could become worse (higher blood pressure and increased blood in the urine).

There were visiting hours twice a day. Usually my mom would come in the morning and both my parents would come after my dad got off his shift as a taxi driver. I was their only child and they thought they were going to lose me. The doctors did not offer any hope.

My mother heard somewhere that garlic could lower blood pressure, so she would bring cloves of raw garlic and chop them down to pill-size for me to swallow. Then I would lie on my bed burping garlic. It did not really bother anyone else, because I was in my bed and only talked to the other kids from a distance. I do not remember if the garlic actually helped or not, but I swallowed a lot of raw garlic.

The other kids were playing and studying, doing art and all kinds of different things, but I had to do everything in my bed. When the nurses caught me out of bed playing with the other kids, they threatened to tie me to the bed to keep me from getting out. After that, I stayed in bed. I was afraid of them.

I had to do all the lessons they sent from school lying down. It was a great frustration not only being in the hospital, but even at the hospital, I was restricted from doing things other kids could do. I could not play with them.

I also had food restrictions. I could not eat anything with salt. They had to prepare my food separately from what other kids were eating and sometimes they would forget to bring my food while they were feeding everyone else. I could not just eat something else; I had to wait until they remembered to bring me my food.

I knew every single nurse and every single doctor by first name. Every morning the nurse would come and draw my blood to check my kidney function. Every day they would draw blood from my arm and every week they would take a blood sample from my finger.

I remember saying to the nurse one day, "I have no more blood to take! You take my blood every day. How long do you think it will take before it runs out?!" She said, "Don't worry, don't worry....we'll give you more blood if you need it." I shouted back, "I don't want somebody else's blood!"

Nevertheless, I did what I was told. I followed instructions. I stayed in bed because I was afraid they would tie me to the bed if I got out.

I had to mark a questionnaire every time I went to the bathroom to report any blood in my urine. They also did a pressure test every day on my inner ankle. They would press the soft tissue on my ankle with their fingers. The skin and muscle were supposed to bounce back, but the finger pressure left a dent that remained imprinted. I did not know that it was an indicator of albumin in my body, but I could see if there was a dent or no dent, so it was something that I could test by myself to see if I was improving. I pressed my own ankle every day looking for the skin to bounce back. Every day, the finger dent stayed.

At the beginning, some of my friends from school would come to visit. Eventually, they stopped coming. They thought I just dropped out of class. A whole summer passed and school started again. I was not there. Three quarters of the school year passed and I still was not at school. I had been in the hospital almost 11 months.

Other kids came and went from the other 29 beds. No one else stayed. I was still there. The doctors did not know what to do with me because they could not get my blood pressure down. There was no change. No improvement.

Another girl with a kidney infection left after one month. I was still there with the same problem. I asked the doctor why she got to go home and I did not. He said that she had recovered, but my body still had not healed from the infection. He did not give me any hope. He never said I was getting better. I was there day after day after day. There was no change. I thought, this is it, I am never going to get out of this hospital ever again. This is the end. I cried myself to sleep many nights.

I celebrated my 10th birthday in the hospital. My mother brought a cake, even though I was not allowed to eat it. It was served to the other children. I did not know if I would ever get out of the hospital or ever see another birthday, but I was afraid I might not. I had the sense that my parents and my doctors felt the same way.

I wanted to get out. I wanted to be able to play with my friends again.

I was still in the bed by the far wall. In April, I got the idea that if I could just move to a bed closer to the door, maybe I would have a chance to leave the hospital. Some of the nurses were very bossy and stern and they would not listen to me, but there was one nurse who was nice. I asked her if I could move closer to the door. She promised that as soon as a bed opened up closer to the door, she would move me.

She was true to her word and as soon as another child left, she moved me to the bed closest to the door. This gave me hope that soon I would be ready to go home. Two weeks later, in May, they decided to let me go home. There was one month of school left. I had to catch up nine months of school in one month, but I passed the exams and was allowed to go to fifth grade.

When I got home from the hospital, I was not allowed to play sports or go out and play with my friends for two months, so my father bought me a TV and put it in my room. It was a black and white TV back then. I would stay up at night watching TV until it went to snow. They did not think about giving me a book to read. They just wanted to entertain me. I was a sad kid, who was not hurt, but could not do anything. I wanted to run. I wanted to play with other kids, but I could not.

They still kept me on a restricted diet when I got home, but no one ever checked to see if I was allergic to anything.

It turned out that I was allergic to things I was eating every day. The severe allergies affected my kidneys and did not allow them to heal from the infection. The doctors did not know that if they had just eliminated gluten and dairy from my diet, my system would have been able to heal. The dairy was inflammatory. In the hospital, they gave me dairy every morning. I refused to drink milk, but I ate cheese and other dairy products, which was maintaining the inflammatory condition in my body.

During the first year after my hospital stay, I still kept getting sick every four or five weeks. They told me I needed to do regular exercise, so I decided to do martial arts. After my first belt test, I went home and told my parents I did not feel good. I had a very high fever. They rushed me to the hospital and it turned out that I had pneumonia. I ended up back in the hospital for a couple weeks and then another two months at home without physical activity. When I finally went back to the karate class, they said they thought I quit, because I disappeared after the test.

This was my life with no consistent health and always in crisis. Every time I showed up at the doctor with a new sore throat, he asked, "How do you keep getting this so bad so fast?" He would give me a new course of antibiotics each time and it would affect my digestion. I stayed in this loop for many years.

I never knew that because I had strong allergies, my immune system was compromised and could not protect me from viruses and bacteria. I know that now. I have learned it. I have mastered it, and I can help other kids. However, as a child, I did not know, and I struggled. I was sick all the time. The joke around my town was that if you want to know if there is a bug going around, you check to see if Aaron is already sick.

When I got out of the hospital, I started experimenting with food. Even at 10 years old, I figured out that something I was eating must have been making me sick, so I tested different things. I tried eliminating dairy from my diet. My stomach never felt good after I ate dairy, so I decided not to eat it for a while. My mother said no, it is good for you, but I argued with her. I insisted it was not good for me and finally got what I wanted. Within a couple of months, I started to get stronger and my body started to function better. I became a new person. However, I still got sick frequently.

It took me longer to make the connection with gluten because it is not always an instant reaction, but can sometimes be a few hours later. It would be several more years until I was in high school before I realized that having a sandwich at lunchtime made my brain foggy later in the afternoon.

When I was 16, I made the connection during Passover, when you do not eat bread. I do not like matzo (thin dry bread Jewish people eat especially at Passover), so I was not eating any wheat products for a week, and I found that my brain was actually functioning better than usual. I had more clarity and could process everything faster. When I looked at my math notes, I could zip right through them. This is when I started testing the idea that bread might be a problem. I would stop eating bread for a few days and then eat bread again for a few days and see how it affected me. This confirmed that it was really affecting my brain function.

I had started eating cheese again, and I found that when I had cheese and bread together it was even worse, weakening my immune system dramatically. So from age 16, when I started to stay away from wheat, my immune system started to get stronger and I stopped being sick every four or five weeks.

***

When I was young, whenever someone asked me what I wanted to be when I grew up, I always said I wanted to be a doctor and work with kids. I never imagined that I would be working with children to clear their allergies in a holistic way. No one in all the years I was sick ever made the connection that my illness could be caused by an allergic reaction. It was only on my own that I began to make that connection. There was a time I ate only eggs for breakfast, lunch and dinner to see if this was what was making me sick. I looked at fruits, beverages, all kinds of things. I knew it was not exercise because I was not doing any exercise. I did not know anything about the mind connection or the role of emotions. However, I knew I ate food every day and I wanted to see if one of them was causing this aggravation. In my mind, the best way to show this was to eat the same thing by itself over and over, then if I had a reaction, it could only be to that thing. I tested by trial and error.

I used to like cheesecake and a goat cheese called labneh but even goat cheese affected me, not just cheese from cows. I tested a variety of things. When I realized that I needed to stay away from all cheeses, my body started to get stronger and stronger.

They say that babies who are breast-fed develop stronger immune systems, but my mother nursed me and I was still very weak, and my immune system did not protect me. Why? Because I developed these allergies. I do not know if my parents had any allergies, because, at the time, no one looked for allergies as a cause of other illnesses.

Chapter 2: The Doctor

"The only true wisdom is in knowing you know nothing."
--Socrates

Even though I wanted to be a doctor as a child, my years training in karate, and later yoga, led me to study to be a physical education teacher in college. The karate, which I had been doing since a few months out of the hospital, was really about using maximum physical force. When I was 16, I started practicing yoga, which was about balance. It really helped me to discipline this power. I started volunteering to teach karate and yoga for a couple hours at a youth center near campus and for a disabled veterans program. I ended up working as a teacher for both karate and yoga full time while I was in college. During that time, I continued learning and competing. I won the national karate championship in Israel and represented Israel in the 1986 Karate World Championship.

When I graduated, I taught PE at middle school and high school levels for two years in Israel before moving to the US, where I continued to teach. I thought that exercise and bodywork was really the solution for health problems, so I decided to study to become a chiropractor. One night I went out for beer and pizza with a chiropractor attending the same seminar. I could not drink beer without falling asleep, and I knew I would have a bad reaction to the wheat and cheese in the pizza. I said to my friend, "You know if I have this pizza and beer, in half an hour I'll be asleep. You'll need to carry me. "He said, "Don't worry. I'll adjust you and you will feel better."

He adjusted me early that night. At 4:30 in the morning, I was carrying him to the hotel, because he had had too much to drink, but I was fine. We had been to multiple bars and I had had a beer and eaten pizza. I did not get the pain in my stomach from the dairy. I did not fall asleep from the wheat and beer. I thought I might still have a reaction the next day, but we were at the seminar for five days, and he adjusted me the same way every day and I was completely fine; my head stayed clear. This is when I realized that if his adjustments could prevent my symptoms in the short term, there might be a way to clear myself from the allergies in the long term. I researched and discovered a technique called NAET.

I started to learn NAET from its creator, Dr. Devi Nambudripad, and worked with my chiropractor friend on myself to clear wheat and dairy. We worked on the treatment little by little every time I saw him over the years, which is much slower than when you do intensive treatment. It got better and better, but did not completely clear until about five years ago. Now I can have cheese, cottage cheese, cheesecake…with no negative effects.

When I started the NAET treatment, I did not even really believe it was possible to clear serious allergies. I thought it would just reduce the symptoms. I started using the treatment on patients in 1995. The first patient I treated was cleared of 62 out of 65 reactions, but was never able to clear the last three.

Over the years, I realized there were deeper layers to the treatment in order to be able to clear it absolutely. We did not do blood analysis back then, but now we have blood tests to show that it is not just the symptoms that disappear. When we implement the whole system of treatments, the body chemistry changes and the antibodies to the allergens disappear.

NAET combines acupuncture meridians, chiropractic treatments, diet, exercise and homeopathic remedies. NAET, on its own, is a marvelous protocol and can clear allergies. It has worked so well for my patients that I became an instructor of the NAET technique. However, sometimes the allergies do not clear as well as expected. Sometimes the technique shows us it will take another thousand treatments to clear the allergy, which could take years. It is not fast enough. I discovered over the years that when we get to this level, if we start to address emotional issues and do reprogramming, we can really address the subconscious of the person. Then the immune system responds differently and can clear the allergies faster.

I had already studied applied kinesiology, which measures muscle strength as a way of identifying structural and other weaknesses in the body. Of all the techniques I have learned, applied kinesiology is the most useful for testing body function.

I went into an in depth study of nutrition so I could also help people with diet and weight loss. I could see direct benefits to patients from chiropractic manipulation and from nutritional changes, but I realized there were mind-body connections I was not addressing. For example, I saw that many times emotions could create allergy symptoms, even when there were no allergies in the blood. Such pseudo or psychosomatic allergies have to be addressed differently.

In order to address these emotional issues, I exposed myself to every technique that I had heard about including NET (Neuro-Emotional Technique), spinal analysis, Zone Healing, Neuro-Linguistic Programming, and other practices. Each technique I studied had fantastic benefits by itself, but I realized that if I combined these great techniques together, I could create the ultimate solution to allergies. Combining complementary techniques makes treatments work faster and deeper.

I realized that for optimum health, we need to help people physically with chiropractic care, specifically through releasing nerves and realigning the body. We need to address diet and nutrition, helping people avoid foods they are allergic to until we clear the allergies and eat the foods that will help strengthen them. Then we need to make the immune system strong enough to be able to keep us healthy and not backfire.

If allergies are not under control, the immune system can react in many ways, such as attacking harmless substances, creating autoimmune diseases or allowing cancerous cells to multiply. We do not know which threats will manage to get past a weakened immune system. However, if we fix the immune system and make it really strong and improve the metabolic function, then the allergies will disappear and the risk of other threats successfully attacking us is reduced. Of course, other things can cause the immune system to weaken. If you are chronically unhappy or sleep-deprived, it can also weaken body function, so you have to address those issues as well for optimal health.

Chapter 3: Why Should I Eliminate, Instead of Just Treat, My Family's Allergies?

"To keep the body in good health is a duty... otherwise we shall not be able to keep our mind strong and clear."
--Buddha

According to the Centers for Disease Control and Prevention 2012-2014 Health Conditions Data, over 35 million children under 18 suffer from respiratory allergy symptoms; 26 million have skin allergies and 12 million have food allergies. (1) These are only the kids who have recognizable allergy symptoms.

If you are an allergy sufferer or have children or other family members who have allergies, you know that avoiding the things you are allergic to, and treating the symptoms, is an ongoing battle. You may feel that keeping the symptoms at bay is a success, and be content with that. Nevertheless, those chronic allergies are actually weakening your entire immune system, making you more susceptible to every other attack on your body.

Your medical doctor may have told you that there is no cure for allergies. I have extensive evidence from my own practice that I will present in the following chapters, which prove not only can you eliminate allergy symptoms permanently, but you can also clear all evidence of allergies from your blood.

When you strengthen your immune system and eliminate even mild allergies, you become healthier overall and are much less likely to succumb to cold and flu viruses or to develop chronic illnesses. When you eliminate more severe, life-threatening allergies, it will create a new freedom in your life that you cannot know when you are on constant alert for an allergic reaction.

The Allergy Free Today Protocol, in the process of treating and clearing allergies, also improves metabolic function, which has the side benefit of eliminating other symptoms not normally seen as allergy related.

Chapter 4: What is the Difference Between Allergy and Sensitivity?

"You cannot depend on your eyes when your imagination is out of focus."
--Mark Twain

According to the National Institute of Allergy and Infectious Diseases, "Approximately 50 percent of Americans have positive skin tests to at least 1 of 10 allergens known to contribute to allergic illness….1 in 20 young children and 1 in 25 adults are allergic to at least one food," and food allergies are on the rise. (2)

In addition to allergies, other allergy-like sensitivities can affect us that are not technically defined as allergies in western medicine. This means that greater than half the population is physically affected.

Both allergies and allergy-like sensitivities are the body's reaction to substances that challenge the body and keep it from functioning correctly.

Allergies

First, let us deal with allergies. We all know when you start sneezing or have breathing issues, or when you start itching, or show a skin reaction such as a rash, hives or acne - that something has happened to cause the immune system to start fighting. The symptoms are a byproduct of the immune system's reaction to the substance that challenges it. This battle of the immune system against what it perceives as invading substances creates a war zone in the body.

In western medicine, the term "allergy" is limited to reactions in the body caused by a specific kind of immunoglobulins, also known as antibodies, called IgE. This is a kind of cell the body creates to battle what it perceives as a threat. Our blood creates some antibodies to fight real infections or diseases, but IgE antibodies are created as an error response to something that is harmless, like pollen. The substance that provokes the response is called an allergen.

Most allergens enter our bodies in two ways, as something that we consume, or something that we breathe. If we react to something we eat or drink, we call it a food allergy. If we react to something we breathe, we call it an environmental allergy. However, we can also react to something that we touch or smell, either environmental or food. Sometimes the energy around a substance is strong enough that we only have to be in its presence to create a reaction in the immune system.

Allergy-Like Sensitivities

When the body has a negative reaction to a substance that cannot be clearly linked to IgE antibodies, it is called an allergy-like sensitivity, a pseudo allergy, or if it is emotion-based, an emotional or psychosomatic allergy.

In addition to respiratory problems and skin reactions, an allergy or allergy-like sensitivity can cause many other symptoms. Sometimes allergies can cause stomach pain or discomfort. Dairy products are the most frequent cause of stomach reactions. Kids will complain of having a tummy ache. It may feel like a sharp knife or just pressure.

Both allergies and allergy-like symptoms can also cause behavioral and cognitive issues. They can slow down the brain process or make us hyperactive.

When you remove allergens from the environment, some kids with ADD and autism can function better, even though they never had any other typical allergy symptoms. This can occur with or without known IgE antibodies in the blood.

The most important thing to understand about both allergy and allergy-like sensitivity is that the body is fighting against a substance that it believes is harmful, but is harmless. If the substance itself were harmful, everyone would react to it. Since most allergens only affect certain people, it is a problem with the body's response mechanism, not with the allergen itself.

When your body reacts to something like a tomato–you get a rash, swollen tongue, or trouble breathing – something in the immune system is not recognizing that this is a safe food most people can eat without getting any reaction. The brain mistakenly identifies it as an enemy.

Allergies consist of two reaction types: instant and delayed. For example, if we eat something that we are allergic to, and within a few minutes to one hour of eating we get hives, this is an instant reaction. However, if the hives result from a meal eaten three days ago, it is a delayed reaction. The symptom is indistinguishable from the instant reaction, but it takes so long to appear, we often don't make the connection.

When we do not recognize the symptoms as a response to an allergy, we can be misdiagnosed and put on medications for other things. Many students diagnosed with ADD cannot control their behavior because of a systemic reaction to something in their diet or surroundings. If the allergic cause can be identified, the problem can be reduced or eliminated by restricting certain foods or changing elements in the environment, helping the kids (or adults) function better.

In hyperactive people, the reaction is often to sugar or a sugar-like product, such as the byproduct of breaking down other food into different sugars. There are 47 different elements of sugar. A person may react to just one, certain ones in combination, or all sugar.

Therefore, the first thing we need to determine is what you or your child is allergic too. The second is how much of that substance it takes to cause a reaction and how severe that allergic reaction is from minor to life threatening. The third is to identify all the different ways the body is reacting.

Chapter 5: History of Allergies and Their Treatment

"A small body of determined spirits fired by an unquenchable faith in their mission can alter the course of history."
--Mahatma Gandhi

The first allergy attack reported in history was of King Menses of Egypt who died from a wasp sting between 3640 and 3300 BC. (3) Many ingredients used in modern medicines for allergies and sinus problems have been in use for over 5000 years in Egypt, China, and the Americas.

Hippocrates (c. 460-377 BC) is considered one of the first physicians to identify a connection between respiratory ailments and the environment. Before then, those in the Greco-roman region usually attributed breathing ailments to sin or demonic possession and treated it with repentance or magic.

Doctors did not make the connection between seasonal sneezing and the environment until the 10th Century in Persia and it took several hundred more years before European physicians caught up with the idea.

Maimonides, a Jewish philosopher and physician from Spain, first made the connection between food and allergies in the 12th century. (4)

Pollen was identified as a cause of respiratory issues in 1859, which led to the first skin scratch test. (3)

In the early 20th Century, research doctors in the United States were testing inoculations on lab animals when they identified "anaphylaxis" as a response to exposure to allergens in milk, egg whites, and other proteins. The term "allergy" was coined in 1906 to describe the body's production of antibodies in response to inoculations that caused asthma symptoms or rash upon a second lower dose inoculation a few days after the first. The connection to seasonal rhinitis, asthma, and certain skin diseases was made a few years later, with histamine first suspected as the cause in 1910.

Around this time, research on immunotherapy led to the development of the allergy shots still used today. Patients receive injections with small amounts of the allergen over time to help their system develop immunity.

The first anti-histamine was released for human use in 1942. (5) Diphenhydramine, more commonly known as Benadryl, was invented in 1943. In 1948, corticosteroids were introduced to treat asthma and allergies. These are still the primary medical treatments for allergies.

The Divergent Field of Clinical Ecology or Environmental Medicine

In 1949, medical doctor and allergy specialist, Theron Randolph, taught at Northwestern University Medical School. He was convinced by taking detailed clinical histories that eating specific foods and exposure to additional environmental factors were responsible for causing illnesses beyond the allergies recognized at the time. He advocated for a more inclusive use of the word allergy beyond just immune response, since he was seeing reactions to foods and environmental substances that the immune system did not mediate.

"I began seeing psychotic and behavioral reactions that were obviously allergic reactions in the broader (non-immunological) sense of the word and began diagnosing hyperactivity in children, and psychotic responses in others as linked with allergy," Randolph said. (6) After sharing his findings with Northwestern faculty, the University dismissed him for his "outlandish ideas."

After leaving Northwestern, he broke with organized medicine to open a series of environmentally controlled clinics where he could treat patients away from contaminating environmental factors. Randolph did extensive clinical research into Multiple Chemical Sensitivity. (7) In 1991, the National Academy of Sciences finally agreed to designate this as a "syndrome," known as Multiple Chemical Sensitivity Syndrome

(MCSS), or more recently Idiopathic Environmental Intolerances (IDEs). It refers to an apparent reaction to chemicals at levels far lower than is normally tolerated by most people.

The Growth of Applied Kinesiology

In the 1930s, physiotherapists, chiropractors, and osteopaths used muscle testing in orthopedic medicine to test motor function of limbs. In 1964, chiropractor George Goodheart, Jr. was using muscle testing in his practice to evaluate the effectiveness of his chiropractic treatments. He made a number of observations connecting muscle function to other health issues beyond the musculoskeletal system and did research to validate his findings. (8) Among other things, he observed connections between muscle strength and allergies, which he reported in a 1969 article, "Allergies in Chiropractic Practice."

In 1976, Goodheart formed the International College of Applied Kinesiology (ICAK), "A system that evaluates structural, chemical and mental aspects of health using manual muscle testing with other standard methods of diagnosis." Applied kinesiology is often used in professional athletics. In fact, George Goodheart was the first official chiropractor to the US Olympic team in 1980.

In 2001, Time magazine listed Goodheart in its Top 100 Alternative Medicine Innovators of the 21st Century. (9) (10)

The Pulse Connection

At the same time George Goodheart was developing applied kinesiology, Arthur F. Coca, MD was discovering a link between an accelerated heart rate and food and other allergies. (11) In the 1920s and 30s, Coca was a professor of immunology at Cornell University in Pennsylvania.

Coca's wife had multiple illnesses that kept her incapacitated for three years. At one point, when Coca commented on his wife's racing heart rate after a treatment, she mentioned that her pulse often sped up after certain meals. They started measuring individual foods to see if there was a connection and found that three foods accelerated her pulse significantly. When she eliminated those foods from her diet, her symptoms went away.

Coca developed a specific protocol for using pulse testing to identify food allergies in his medical practice. He reported his findings and methodology in the book, *The Pulse Test* (1956). (11)

Ongoing Research Related to Allergy Treatment

Since the 1980s, starting with scientists at the National Institute of Health and the Massachusetts Institute of Technology, molecular biologists, neuroanatomists and neuroscientists have been increasing the body of knowledge proving how thoughts and emotions affect chemical and electrical signals in the body. (12) This supports the need to treat the thoughts and emotions as well as the physical systems involved in allergies.

Since the late 1990s, MRI technology has confirmed that the meridians used in Oriental Medicine align with their corresponding organs and systems. (13) (14) These meridians are used in the Allergy Free Today Protocol.

Chapter 6: The Difference between the Medical and Holistic Approach to Allergies

"The fundamental law of nature is that all force must be kept in balance."

--Thomas Edison

In general, three elements influence the health of our bodies:

1. We can have physical injuries to our bodies, like a trauma or repetitive motion damage.
2. We can have organic attacks such as viruses, bacteria, fungi, or parasites – anything that invokes a chemical response in the body. Allergies fall into this category, since the body does not recognize the allergens and reacts as if it is under attack.
3. The third level is the emotional level, or autosuggestion. This is where our own self-talk and belief system can cause us to become sick or can also help us to regain health. It involves emotional and psychological elements.

The Medical Approach

The medical approach deals primarily with treating illness and injuries. Medical doctors study the pathology of diseases in order to treat symptoms. The holistic approach focuses more on optimal wellness. It looks at creating balance in the body so that the immune system is strong enough to fight off any threats and heal injuries.

Medical doctors are experts in a few areas. One of them is treating the body with chemicals. They can prescribe pharmaceutical chemicals, like antihistamines to shut down symptoms in the body. This works faster than anything else for treating many symptoms. It often does not fix the problem, but the person feels better. Many times, we need to feel better or eliminate symptoms to avoid going into a crisis state. The problem is that when we sacrifice our health to feel better in the short term, we are setting ourselves up for long term problems.

Medical doctors are also the only ones who have surgery as a tool for some things, but this is not applicable to allergy treatment. For allergies, the primary benefit of a medical doctor is the ability to prescribe pharmaceutical drugs for the symptoms.

In the United States, medical doctors also have the advantage of being able to order a full array of lab tests including skin tests and blood analysis, and have them at least partially covered by insurance. Most insurance companies will not cover the same tests when ordered by a naturopathic doctor or other holistic practitioner.

Although medical doctors have advanced tools for diagnosis, their treatment options are limited primarily to prescribing antihistamines for environmental allergies, or recommending you stay away from foods you are allergic to.

One additional treatment option for medical doctors is to use immunotherapy. This can be in the form of regular shots or drops containing the allergen. It is initially administered multiple times a week with reduced frequency over a period of years to help the body build a tolerance to the allergen. This can reduce the symptoms for some people who do not respond well to antihistamines or have year-round allergies. Aside from the fact that most people don't want to go through getting shots multiple times a week for an extended period, this kind of pharmaceutical immunotherapy doesn't eliminate the allergy from the blood. It just reduces the symptoms and reactions.

The Holistic Approach

The holistic approach addresses body-mind communication and prioritizes wellness and balance. Practitioners treat the body in a variety of ways.

Chiropractors do manipulation to improve the body's alignment and allow the nervous system to function effectively. Sometimes this manipulation can change reactions to asthma conditions and allergies.

Acupuncture uses needles to stimulate the nervous system; changing the electric impulses in the body to overcome allergies. Acupuncturists also use different herbs that you smell, taste or take. Although acupuncturists have been treating allergies with positive results and minimal side effects since ancient times, acupuncture only relieves the symptoms and does not clear them permanently.

Naturopaths use all kinds of homeopathic remedies, herbs, nutritional supplements and essential oils. They use combinations and different formulas to help the body overcome allergies by strengthening the immune system or correcting the gut, which is the mother of the immune system. They approach more areas and have a greater variety of treatment methods to deal with allergies.

The Allergy Free Today Protocol uses the same testing method as medical doctors – a very thorough blood analysis. Once we identify the allergies, the treatment includes changing the energy in the body and correcting the nervous system function with homeopathic support and then reprogramming the mind. We get excellent results. When we retest the patient after treatment, we see in the majority of patients that the allergic response in the blood is reduced or eliminated completely.

One of my young patients came to me with allergies to peanuts, walnuts, white rice, and shrimp at anaphylactic level four and above. When we retested him after one year, he was down to zero reaction in everything except peanuts, which was down to Class 1. The peanut allergy was also reduced from an allergic response to six of seven proteins in peanuts, to being allergic to just one of the seven proteins. He no longer has any apparent reaction to peanuts and can safely be exposed to them. The mother no longer needs to carry an EpiPen everywhere.

If you suspect you have allergies and want to improve your health, and you have medical insurance, I recommend that you approach an allergy doctor for blood tests for food, vitamin, and environmental allergies. If you have many allergies, it may be necessary to test up to 450 different substances. The insurance company is more likely to approve more extensive testing from an allergy specialist than from a primary care doctor. Once results are in hand, find a holistic practitioner like myself to help eliminate these allergies permanently. After the treatment is finished, I recommend going back to the medical doctor to do another test to make sure everything is 100% clear.

If you do not have insurance that would cover the full allergy panel, some holistic practitioners may be able to order the tests for less than the cash rate your medical doctor will charge.

Chapter 7: The Systems Involved in Correcting Allergies

"The higher your energy level, the more efficient your body. The more efficient your body, the better you feel."
--Anthony Robbins

The four systems involved in correcting allergies are the immune system, nervous system, endocrine system, and digestive system. The brain sends messages chemically through the endocrine system, electrically through the nervous system, and supports the immune system nutritionally through the digestive system. All of the systems are interactive, communicating with each other all of the time.

The Immune System

The immune system is the warrior. It protects us from inside by investigating and healing any system that is not working properly. Viruses and bacteria are attempting to get inside our system all the time. We are exposed to them constantly, but most of the time they do not succeed because the immune system keeps them out. In addition to viruses and bacteria, parasites, fungi, toxins, worms, and other things can attack our system. Our body learns to deal with them and to fight them to protect us. Of course, in higher doses of exposure they can overcome and challenge the body, to the extent that we get sick even with a strong immune system.

The immune system also protects us from errors in cell duplication. It is like the police force monitoring the regeneration of 500 million new cells every day and killing any cell that is not a perfect match for your DNA. Some of our cells last a lifetime, but most of them last from a few days to a few months. Every single cell needs to be tested, and if it is not a match, the immune system takes it aside and kills it so it does not become cancer or create autoimmune diseases.

The Endocrine System

The endocrine system works chemically. It includes the pineal gland, pituitary gland, pancreas, ovaries, testes, thyroid gland, parathyroid gland, hypothalamus, gastrointestinal tract, and adrenal glands that secrete hormones in the circulatory system, which regulates metabolism, sleep, mood, and other major functions of the body.

The hypothalamus is the control center for all the other organs of the endocrine system. The endocrine system sends chemical signals that can impact the body for a few hours up to several weeks.

In addition to the specialized endocrine organs mentioned above, other parts of the body, such as bone, kidney, liver, heart, and gonads, can also participate in endocrine functions by secreting hormones.

The Brain and the Nervous System

The nervous system, operated by the brain, is the electric system that sends and receives electrical charges throughout your body. It is the largest system communicating messages between the brain and the cells of the body, controlling what your body does.

The nervous system is a unique system because there are a huge number of wires, which send messages with a very low impulse - one millionth of a volt. The nervous system of the average adult contains over 45 miles of nerve fibers. (15) If the brain identifies something as a danger, it immediately sends a message to the immune system.

Allergy is an error in the brain – a flaw in the master controller of the nervous system – where it identifies something as a danger that is actually harmless. Although medical science recognizes this as an error, they have not identified a medical treatment to correct this error.

The brain receives 11 million bits of data from your five senses, and 70 million bits of data from the rest of your body every second. (16) (17) When the communication within the body is not very good, the brain may not receive the correct message or may receive it and not respond or ignore it completely. Even if the immune system says the substance is safe, the brain may miss the message and attack anyway.

The Digestive System

The digestive system is a group of organs working together to convert food into energy and basic nutrients to feed the entire body. Digestion involves the breakdown of food into smaller and smaller components, until they can be absorbed and assimilated into the body.

What is a little tricky to understand is that most of the work of the digestive system happens outside the body – even though it is happening within the interior of the body. The stomach and intestines are like a hollow hose or tunnel through the body. The water is not part of the hose, even though it goes through it, and the car driving through the tunnel is not part of the mountain. Whatever is inside the stomach is outside the body, not incorporated into it. The digestive system uses enzymes to break down food, extract the nutrients and pass them through the walls of the intestines into the body as the food passes through the hose on its way back out.

Whatever gets broken down correctly can be absorbed and passed into the blood. From the blood, it goes to the liver. This is the pharmaceutical part of our body. It cleans out toxins and directs the nutrients to build whatever they need to construct. The liver is the only organ that can regenerate itself after partial removal.

Inside the hose that goes through us, we live in harmony with Candida and a variety of bacteria that we refer to as good bacteria. When they interact with food and break it down, they create specific enzymes and extract vitamins that are beneficial to us. We work together in a cooperative partnership. There are more good bugs inside the intestines of each of us than there are people on the planet. There are also good bacteria that live on our skin and help protect us on the outside.

The first stop in the digestive system is our mouth, where chewing our food starts producing the digestive enzymes that will process the food. The next stop is the stomach, which creates a very acidic environment.

This stomach acid does two major things. First, it breaks down protein. Protein is tough and needs a very acidic environment with low PH to break it down effectively. Second, the acidity of the stomach can help kill invaders. Stomach acid is like the cleaning crew that is the first defense in cleaning up toxins that can harm us.

If the invaders survive the stomach, they pass through to the intestines, a very high PH environment that nourishes them and where viruses can grow rapidly. Chewing your food really well helps the stomach do its job of killing those viruses and bacteria before they can get to the intestine.

Most of the enzymes required for digestion are triggered by the endocrine system, secreted by the pancreas and passed into the small intestine, where the nutrients are broken down into small enough molecules to be absorbed through the walls of the intestine into the blood stream. The length of the entire human intestine is 25 to 28 feet with multiple layers of tissue on the inside, so there is a lot of surface area to absorb nutrients – about the surface area of a tennis court if you stretched out all the layers.

The nervous system controls the muscle contractions that helps move food through the length of your small and large intestines. There are different tiny structures on the inner surface of the intestines to absorb different kinds of nutrients. The three different sections of the small intestine also absorb different nutrients into the bloodstream. The majority of nutrients are absorbed in the middle section of the small intestine, but iron is absorbed in the upper section and B12 in the lowest section. If any section is surgically removed, damaged or blocked, then your body cannot absorb those nutrients from food.

A few substances are more easily absorbed and can even start being absorbed in the stomach. Alcohol is one example that starts breaking down and being absorbed in the stomach so it affects the blood right away, which is why alcohol can take effect so quickly.

We say that the intestine is the father and mother of the immune system. If your intestine is not functioning very well, the chances of your immune system being able to support you is not very good. If the intestinal walls are not working very well because they are never cleaned, and they are not absorbing nutrients properly, your immune system does not have the necessary tools to function. The immune system is the most important system to protect us, but it is very fragile and many different things can weaken it.

In addition to insufficient nutrient absorption, another item that commonly affects the immune system is excessive sugar consumption. For example, drinking one can of soda, which contains over nine teaspoons of sugar, can reduce the body's immune function by 50% for four to six hours. During that four to six hour period, we are more vulnerable to getting sick. If allergies are already taxing your immune system, and then you drink soda on top of that, the allergic reaction may be more severe when you are exposed to allergens.

Most of us are diligent about cleaning the outside of our bodies daily. The digestive system that passes nutrients through our body also benefits from a thorough cleanse every four to six months. This is why, after balancing the metabolic function, we do a detox protocol to cleanse the intestine and eliminate anything that should not be there. Once cleared, everything will work better. Nutrients will absorb better and the immune system will get the support it needs to function optimally.

These four systems and the communications between them functions 24 hours a day. The protocol I created is a combination of ten treatment methods that deal with all four systems. It balances the body's basic metabolic functions including hormones; cleanses and balance the digestive system; overcomes nervous system errors; and resets the brain, so that the brain will no longer misidentify the allergen, and no longer produce symptoms ever again. That is the Allergy Free Today Protocol.

Chapter 8: Other Stressors that Impact Your Immune Response

"Breathe. Let go. And remind yourself that this very moment is the only one you know you have for sure."

--Oprah Winfrey

Other stressors can affect the immune system and have an indirect relationship to allergies. For example, today's food contains unnecessary chemicals designed to stimulate the sensory system and tempt excessive consumption. Some companies research chemicals to improve flavor and stimulate eating more of their product, seeing product addiction as an effective marketing strategy. (18) Researchers found that Oreo cookies cause a similar brain response to cocaine. (19) Other companies use genetic modification without fully realizing the effect it could have on the long-term health of our bodies.

We cannot avoid these products completely, so it's in our best interest to keep our immune system operating at peak performance. Three chemically altered food classifications significantly compromise our immune systems: genetically modified organisms (GMO), saturated fats, and processed sugars.

If you ingest GMO foods, such as chips cooked in cottonseed oil or a chemically enhanced food, you bombard your immune system. (20)

If you consume saturated fats (concealed in many foods), it promotes both inflammatory and histamine reactions in your body. In addition, the body takes close to 60 days to break it down and clear the system. Otherwise, unsaturated fats take two weeks. (20)

If you eat or drink products made with processed sugars, such as a can of soda (~ 7 to 10 tsp/~15 grams sugar), you challenge the immune system, decreasing its function up to 50% for four to six hours.

Some things that are harmless or even helpful in small doses can stress the system. For example, 20 minutes of sun every day benefits the skin and the rest of the body while improving the immune system through natural vitamin D absorption. Yet extended **sun exposure** causes your body to go into overdrive. It produces excess melanin to protect the skin, but it cannot produce it fast enough, so you burn. The ultraviolet light from the sun can also cause changes to your DNA under the skin's surface, prematurely aging your skin. (21)

Your strong immune system can fight off altered DNA cells, but if your system is compromised, they can replicate unhindered. Over time, DNA damage from the sun can contribute to skin cancers, including deadly melanoma. (22) If your immune system is busy fighting DNA-altering sun damage, it reduces available resources for fighting other intruders.

Wound healing also pulls immune response away from infection fighting. A stressed immune system – especially one that has been under long-term stress from allergies or other illnesses – starts fighting new cells created in healing so the body has a harder time healing wounds and mending broken bones. (23)

Traumatic injuries disrupt the immune system and predisposes patients to opportunistic infections and inflammatory complications. (24) When the immune system is busy healing a wound, it leaves the body more susceptible to infections and viruses.

Emotional Stressors weaken the immune system. Stressfūl events that last a few minutes or hours, and are quickly forgotten, do not present problems. However, chronic stress, pain, or heightened adrenaline sustainment - regardless of type: emotional or physical - can weaken the immune system. (23) (25)

Lack of sleep is one of the most common contributors to immune system reduction. Sleep is the time when our immune system is most productive. Without good quality sleep, your immune cells do not have time to function properly. When we sleep, our bodies remove toxins and regulate hormones to keep our systems in balance. For example, it takes the full eight-hour sleep cycle for the pancreas to maintain the body's daily supply of insulin. (26)

You will find many sources debunking the idea that you can catch a cold from being cold. However, research now shows that cold suppresses the immune system, so you are more susceptible to a virus or bacteria that your body might otherwise be able to fight off.

Given the number of factors that affect the immune system, it is important to reduce these aforementioned stressors in order to build the immune system up as we work on reinforcing the metabolic functions.

Chapter 9: Symptoms of Allergies

"Start where you are. Use what you have. Do what you can."

--Arthur Ashe

As we discussed in Chapter Three, the most common allergic symptoms that people are aware of are skin conditions and respiratory issues.

Skin conditions may include eczema, psoriasis, rash, hives, or other bumps. Respiratory issues include sinus congestion, runny nose, sneezing, itchy, watery eyes, or general difficulty breathing. These are the most common symptoms that most people recognize as allergic reactions.

However, allergies can affect us in many ways that we do not even think of as allergies. They may manifest as behavioral issues that look like ADD or ADHD. These symptoms can be a result of food or environmental allergies. We do not know why autism symptoms can sometimes be a reaction to even a very mild allergy, but we know that when we eliminate the allergies, one can function better and can communicate better. Others have the same allergies that show up even more severely in their blood, but it does not affect their communication or behavior at all.

Some allergy symptoms are interpreted as unrelated. For example, asthma can be a strong allergic reaction to the environment, but is sometimes treated as a completely independent illness. When we start to clear the allergies, the patient gradually reduces and eventually eliminates the need for an inhaler. We slowly make their body strong enough so he or she no longer needs medication.

I used to be seriously allergic to dairy and gluten, primarily wheat. The dairy would create major pain and discomfort in my intestine and abdomen. I would get the pain right away; it felt like someone was stabbing me with a knife and twisting it all the time. I was in a lot of pain. Usually the pain would last six to 48 hours and then it would go away. I did not know growing up that I had an allergy. I was not even aware that allergies existed, but I knew that when I avoided certain foods, I felt better. Therefore, I tried for most of my life to avoid dairy – no milk, no cheese, nothing. Today I can eat dairy with no problem. No reaction.

I was also allergic to wheat, which created an entirely different reaction. It affected my thought process. It slowed down my thinking. Suddenly I could not put words together in sentences or paragraphs. If someone asked me a question, even when I knew the answer, I could not recall the answer. It affected me more mentally than anything else did.

When I was growing up and going to school, the worst thing for me was having a cheese sandwich before math class. I could not do the math because my brain process had slowed down dramatically, and I had a stomachache. With time, I started to realize that wheat is actually an issue for me, so I started to eat less and less wheat. Suddenly when I went to college, and I completely stayed away from dairy and wheat, I could think clearly and process things very well.

Today I am not allergic to either one of them. I can even have pizza, which has both dairy and wheat, with no reaction. I can process, think, analyze and have no pain and no discomfort. However, this took years of not knowing, before I learned how to clear the issues permanently.

The table on the next page is a partial list of symptoms that have been relieved by addressing underlying allergies and allergy-like sensitivities.

A Partial list of conditions that can be directly or indirectly related to allergies and non-allergy sensitivities:

ALLERGIES	DISEASES	OTHER
Chemicals	Acne	ADD/ADHD
Chemotherapy	Arthritis	Anxiety
Clothing	Asthma	Autism
Cold	Autoimmune	Bad Breath
Computer	Colds	Constipation
Cosmetics	Blood Pressure	Depression
Dairy Products	Bronchitis	Dry Eyes
Dust	Candida/Yeast	Dyslexia
Foods	Chronic Fatigue	Flatulence
Fungus	Colitis	Food Cravings
Heat	Cough	Hair Loss
Latex	Diarrhea	Itching
Mold	Ear Infections	Hemorrhoids
Peanuts	Eating Disorders	Hives
Penicillin	Eczema	Hyperactivity
Pets & Animals	Fibromyalgia	Indigestion
Plastics	Gallstones	Insomnia
Pollen	Gout	Knee Pain
Prescription Drugs	Hay Fever	Migraines
Radiation	Headaches	Mood Swings
Shellfish	Heart Problems	Morning
The Sun	Herpes	Sickness
	Hormone Imbalances	Motion Sickness
Your Children	Hypoglycemia	Nervous
Your Co-Workers	Infections	Stomach
Your Parents	Irritable Bowel Syndrome	Night Sweats
Your Spouse	Kidney Disease	Overeating
	Leaky Gut	O.C.D.
ADDICTIONS:	Lupus	Phobias
Smoking	Post Nasal Drip	Poor Appetite
Alcohol	Psoriasis	Poor Memory
Carbohydrates	Shingles	PMS
Coffee	Sinusitis	Vertigo
Drugs		Vision Problems
Food		Weight Issues

Chapter 10: Testing for Allergies

"Knowledge is power. Information is liberating."
--Kofi Annan

In general, we have two kinds of medical tests and a number of self-tests for allergies.

The Allergy Skin Test

A skin test is where we actually scratch the body with the allergen to see if the body will react. If the body reacts, the reaction is measured from Class 1 to Class 4, depending on how big of a welt it creates. Class 4 is very severe. It means an anaphylactic reaction. Class 1 has very little reaction, with zero being no reaction. If there is no reaction at all, it means the body does not have sensitivity to this allergen. Aside from the fact that having your skin pricked repeatedly and itching is unpleasant, the skin test also runs the risk of inducing a severe reaction.

Blood Tests for Allergies

We can also test for allergies by testing the blood for antibodies to specific allergens. When we test the blood, we can see even more information. Blood tests can measure four different factors: IgA, IgE, IgG and IgM.

IgM is for the mucus layer of the abdomen that shows whether the body is allergic to gluten or any kind of grain. For this test, we usually expose the patient to grain within 24 hours before the test to create the reaction so it can be measured.

IgG tests non-allergy sensitivities.

IgE is the most important test because it measures the body's antibodies to allergens in six levels of severity instead of just four, and you can see variation within each class. This range within each class gives us a lot more information to understand what is going on in the body. It can tell us clearly, for example, if the body has any allergies Class 4 and above. Class 4, even at the lowest level, is anaphylactic and is life threatening, which requires you to carry an EpiPen at all times to be able to intervene immediately in case of a severe reaction. If it is Class 5 or 6, you should completely avoid the specific antigen that you are allergic to. You have to be constantly vigilant, knowing that you can unexpectedly be exposed to the allergen at any time, so you cannot go anywhere without the EpiPen.

Because of the extra detail in the blood test, compared to the skin test, you can see if a patient moves from a high Class 4 to a low Class 4, for example, and then from a low Class 4 to a high Class 3. As a first step, we want to take them to Class 3 and lower, which is the difference between having to carry an EpiPen wherever you go, and not needing the EpiPen. The ultimate goal is to put everybody in Class 0 or between zero and one so that after treatment, they will not react to anything, and they will be able to function very well. They will be able to eat or be exposed to the allergens without having a reaction. This is the unique approach of Allergy Free Today.

The Pulse Test

The Pulse Test, created by Dr. Arthur Coca, is a test you can do yourself to confirm exposure to allergens. You start by checking your resting pulse in the morning, just after waking up, three days in a row to establish a baseline resting heart rate. There are smartphone apps that can measure your pulse. Once you have a baseline for your normal resting heart rate, when you eat, wait fifteen minutes and take your pulse. If it varies from the pulse baseline more than six counts, this indicates allergen exposure. (11)

Rib Test Point

There is a histamine reflex point on your lower right rib that you can test with your fingers to see if you are having an allergy reaction. Pain at this point indicates exposure to allergens that are creating a histamine reaction. (See Resources at the end of this book.)

Chapter 11: Diet to Eliminate Allergies

"Tell me what you eat, and I will tell you who you are."

--Jean Anthelme Brillat-Savarin

The pulse test is the first step towards allergy elimination at home. It requires multiple pulse measurements to detect allergy exposure incidents.

When you suspect that you have allergies because of the pulse test results – increased pulse of five or more above baseline – you can trace which food item(s) caused it.

You can test one specific food item for a reaction. To begin this process, establish the same meal – the same set of food items – for breakfast, lunch and dinner. Eat the same meal three times a day for three days, totaling nine meals. After every meal, wait fifteen minutes and check your pulse. Whatever we eat departs our body around four days later. If you do not have a pulse rate increase of more than five beats after waiting fifteen minutes after each meal, for nine meals in a row, the food items in this meal are not allergens and are safe to eat. They become your baseline. If you include a new item in nine consecutive meals with no reaction (measure pulse after each meal as before), the new item is safe. If there is a reaction, you are allergic to this food.

For example, let us say you want to test for an allergy to cucumber. (Ground rule: if there has been no prior reaction to these, you can assume chicken and white rice are safe base foods.) You eat chicken, rice, and cucumber for nine meals in a row for breakfast, lunch, and dinner – with no other foods or snacks in between. If after nine meals, you see no symptoms of any kind, we can add cucumber to the safe list and add another food to the meal plan. We may try carrots, then tomatoes, then peppers, then add beef or fish, different kinds of fish, maybe pasta. With pasta and anything else that is processed, you need to make sure you use the same brand for all nine meals.

I tested one patient for tomatoes and she was fine, but when we tested for tomato sauce, she had a reaction. We tested four more brands of tomato sauce, but she only reacted to the first one.

If any symptom happens after any of the nine meals, you stop it for a few days and then try it again. If you get the same symptom again, add this to the list of things to avoid. Slowly through this diet, we build a foundation of food we can eat without allergies.

Soft drinks, juices, and other beverages can also trigger allergens. This means that after only having water, you might add apple juice (or whatever beverage you prefer) to your nine consecutive meals. If your pulse exceeds six counts above normal after any one of the nine meals, you can eliminate that from your diet. Stop eating it if you have a reaction even once. If you find that you are allergic to 20 to 30 foods that are processed foods, no big deal; just avoid them. However, if they are natural, non-GMO foods like cucumbers, tomatoes, apples, or bananas (to name a few), then it is a serious allergy. We need to address it much faster to correct it, because no reaction of any kind should result from naturally occurring foods.

If you have allergies to bread, pasta, gluten, and other processed starch, we should address it and eliminate it, but it is not as urgent as the natural foods. If you want to test something you do not like, just take two bites. Do not force too much upon yourself or your child because it can create an emotional reaction. Keep up the two bites for nine meals.

Make the "good list" as rich as possible, so that you have more and more foods that are safe to eat. You use the same process for drinks if you want to drink different juices or sodas. Not that sodas or juices are healthy, but it is better that you test them to make sure they are not actually causing harm. You can also compare store-bought orange juice to juice you squeeze at home to see if there is a difference in reaction.

Although you can use this method to find foods to simply avoid, if you have a lot of food sensitivities, avoiding them all can lead to poor nutrition. We use this diet to identify the problem foods, and then we clear them one by one until you are not allergic to any of them.

Chapter 12: Emotional Allergies

"The thing you fear most has no power. Your fear of it is what has the power."
--Oprah Winfrey

When we refer to emotional allergies, we are talking about cases where patients have symptoms in response to specific products or substances, but have no antibodies in their blood to explain the reaction. Just like normal allergies, emotionally induced allergic reactions can be in response to food or environmental factors, and exposure can result from consumption, breathing, touching, smelling, or being in the proximity of the trigger substance.

What is going on is something called emotional behavior (also known as psychosomatic symptoms). This is when our body develops a physical response as a reaction to a bad experience. It can be very involved to track down the source of the problem, but we try to make it as simple, gentle, and painless to the patient as possible.

For example, I had a patient who had a severe reaction to strawberries, but there was no IgE or IgG reaction in the blood. There were, however, clear skin and behavioral symptoms triggered by strawberries. A contradiction between the blood results and the body's reaction to the strawberries indicated that there might be an emotional cause for the symptoms.

When he first came to my office and we did the metabolic tests, he did show some metabolic weaknesses, so I treated him for those to improve body function first. Then we did the blood test for strawberries. His test did not show an allergy to strawberries. We did the skin test. No reaction. We had to start looking for emotional causes. I asked his mother if there was any emotional issue related to strawberries, and it took time and a lot of discussion before the mother remembered an incident involving strawberry pie.

My patient was a ten-year-old boy who, years earlier, had failed a test at school. He had to take the test home and get it signed by his parents. When he showed it to his mom and asked her to sign it, she said no, that she needed to show it to his dad. The dad came home from work that evening and they all sat down to dinner together. All through dinner, the son waited for his mother to tell his father, but she did not say anything. He was very nervous about what his father would say. For dessert, the mother served strawberry pie. Then she finally told her husband that their son had failed the test and was not doing well at school.

The father was probably very tired and was not mentally prepared to respond constructively. He started screaming at his wife. "I'm working and supporting this family. It is your responsibility to take care of the kid and help him with his schoolwork! It's your fault!" She yelled back, "Why is it my fault?" and they kept fighting back and forth.

They never addressed the son or talked to him about it. He just sat at the table eating his pie. He suddenly stood up from the table and ran to the bathroom to throw up everything he had just eaten. They stopped fighting to check on him, make sure he was okay, and take care of him.

Life went on and this story was completely forgotten, but that incident created a connection in his body between what he ate and the emotional response to that fight. Every time he ate strawberries, his subconscious learned to react severely. He did not throw up. His mouth and tongue would swell up and he would develop a rash around his mouth as if it were a normal allergen-induced reaction, but there were no antibodies in his blood. This was an entirely emotional response.

Once we identified the emotional trigger, we did NET (Neuro-Emotional Technique), the emotional release technique that we do for allergies related to emotions, and we found a correlation. We did a treatment to clear the emotion connected to the incident. Then we worked on strawberries.

I asked the mother to bring me strawberries. We treated him with fresh strawberries using NAET and NET. After that treatment, he overcame his aversion to strawberries, but he did not strawberry pie. Therefore, I had the mother bring strawberry pie and we treated him again with the pie. We also did reprogramming to give his subconscious a different positive message about strawberries and strawberry pie, so his body would function optimally and not be triggered by emotional responses in the future. After these treatments, he no longer had any reaction to strawberries. Today he is 16 and doing great.

A woman came to my office for treatment. One day she asked if I could help her husband who was having migraines every day. When I met the husband, we tried to figure out why he was getting the migraines.

He said he came home every day from work and would go straight to the kitchen to heat up some water for tea. He said he would instantly get a migraine. Sometimes he did not even drink the tea, but within an hour of arriving home, he would get a migraine.

We tested the tea, and it was not the tea. We tested other things from the kitchen and the bedroom. Nothing there. We tested the clothes. Nothing. Then I realized the most painful thing possible was that he was allergic to his wife. Therefore, I brought both of them in the office to treat both of them, and then the wife had to stay away from the husband for 25 hours. After the treatment, his headaches disappeared and never came back.

Another example of an emotional allergy is something that is common with autistic kids. Most autistic kids have an allergy-like reaction to one or both parents. One of the first things we do with autistic kids is to clear the relationship with the parent who is the primary caregiver. It is not always the primary caregiver, but often it is.

It is a challenge for families. We usually do the treatment on Fridays, when the parent gets off work. During the treatment, the child and the parent have to stay in physical contact for 20 minutes, which can be really challenging for an autistic child. Then the parent has to stay away from the child completely with no contact for 25 hours, just as we do for a food allergy.

This treatment completely changes the relationship between parent and child and opens the door for children to respond better to their ongoing allergy treatment. Some kids initially do not even participate in the treatment. After we do this, they become more cooperative. For this treatment, we need both parents, or for single parents, a second responsible adult to care for the child for 25 hours.

Emotional Intervention and Reprogramming

Emotional intervention is the last phase of treatment. If a person is allergic to a specific food, first we address the metabolic function, and then we do a blood analysis and treat the specific food. It does not matter if we clear the allergy physically or not. Even if it shows cleared in the blood and immediate symptoms, we want to make sure that the brain does not react and that no emotional trigger exists that would cause the symptoms to come back in the future.

I test for emotional factors for every single allergy, but there are different ways to get at emotional issues. In the reprogramming phase, I ask patients to use their imagination to make sure they are strong and healthy and that the immune system is functioning well, not reacting to anything it shouldn't react to, but reacting to things when it needs to react. We do not want to shut down the immune system so it does not react when there is really something it needs to eliminate.

For example, if you are allergic to cucumbers, we want to clear the allergic reaction to them, but if you eat a cucumber contaminated with bacteria that is dangerous, we want your immune system to be able to react to the bacteria, not to the cucumber.

The closing treatment is always the reprogramming, regardless of whether it is an environmental issue or an allergy to food. We reprogram the immune system to do the right job. The reprogramming gives the command for the immune system to execute its mission perfectly to protect us from real environmental risks or internal duplication errors.

Health is about balance, both physically and emotionally.

Chapter 13: What is the Allergy Free Today Protocol?

"The way to get started is to quit talking and begin doing."
--Walt Disney

The Stop Allergy Now Protocol incorporates several disciplines such as allopathy, chiropractic, acupressure, kinesiology, nutrition, homeopathic, and psychological solutions (body-mind connection). The protocol takes patients through the following phases of treatment:

1. Determine if you have allergies with the self-testing methods in Chapter 9.
2. Avoid everything that tests positive (pulse increase of six or more).
3. Improve the metabolic function.
4. Clean the body systems (detoxification program).
5. Test the blood for food and environmental allergies, and treat the individual foods and environmental substances to eliminate allergies one by one.
6. Take herbal and nutritional supplements for the four systems: nervous, immune, digestive, and endocrine.

7. Identify any emotional blockage and replace with supportive self-messages, reprogramming the unconscious mind for optimal health.

First, we want to improve the body's metabolic function. This is the body's basic engine or operating system. If I ask you what your car needs to operate, you would tell me it needs gas, oil, and fluids in specific locations like brake fluid and transmission fluid. It needs water and coolant. It needs air, and its lights and computer run on electricity. If we change one element – if we decrease the electricity or use too much air or not enough fluid – the car will not run very well. It might even break down.

The body works the same way. It needs vitamins, minerals, sugars, proteins, oils (fatty acids), and carbohydrates. It converts everything to acids and bases from the foods we eat, and communicates through hormonal and electrical signals. This is the body's basic engine operating system.

The brain communicates through the endocrine system biochemically via hormones and sends electrical signals through the nervous system.

Thus, when you improve the body's metabolic system, you take it from functioning okay, to running like a racecar on pure fuel with a perfectly tuned transmission and everything running smoothly, in top working order, with the least possible effort. This is the idea behind correcting the body's metabolic function.

We use several techniques, described below, to fine-tune the metabolic function. After the metabolic function improves, the system works better. Additionally, if the system works better, some of the errors in the brain that we call allergies disappear on their own. The next step, before we clear the allergies, is to make sure that all the lines of communication are clean. We use a detox program to help the body in this process. This is a 10-day high-power diet designed to pile on nutrients while clearing toxins.

Next, we move on to clearing environmental or food allergies, starting with whichever category seems to be causing the most severe symptoms or has the highest IgE levels in the blood. Each person gets a customized protocol depending on their specific allergies. Within the category of food or environment, we start with the mild allergies that usually clear in one treatment. This frees up immune resources to tackle the more severe allergies in that category. If environmental allergies are more severe, we remove allergies to things that are in the environment, like pollen, dust, flowers, trees, or chemicals – whatever element(s) in the environment are challenging the body. Then we work on food.

The final step is to clear all the emotional negativity that holds us back and reprogram the brain to correct those errors. An error in the brain is like an error in a computer program that causes a software glitch. If you go to the programmer and point out the mistake, he can correct the mistake, and the error that crashed the computer or hung up the program clears. However, we do not just want to patch the software, we want to install a better program so the brain can function at its highest capacity.

The brain controls many different things, most of them at an unconscious level we don't perceive. All emotions, positive and negative, derive from and reside in the limbic system of the brain. If we remove the negative emotions and replace them with positive emotions, we reprogram the person to become healthy and allergy-free for life.

To do the reprogramming, we talk in advance about what we want to accomplish, then put you in relaxation mode and talk you through imaginary scenarios – independent of the past, present, or future reality. We use the power of imagination to vividly create situations that reprogram what we want. We record this, and when you listen to the suggestions repeatedly in a relaxed state, they become part of you. It is like learning a new skill. We reprogram health instead of sickness. We program success instead of failure. We program a powerful immune system to fight whatever it needs to – attacking the right things, not the wrong things – keeping the immune system neutral to anything that is not a real threat.

The reprogramming usually takes a few months. We have a few different messages that we do. You listen to them twice a day while awake for one to four weeks, and consciously agree with everything in each statement. If you do not agree, we change it.

Then we alternate messages until we finish all the reprogramming. You leave here very, very happy.

I use homeopathic remedies to support the entire process, helping the nervous system overcome resistance and increase metabolic function. It also helps increase the system's ability to fight allergies to food or environmental elements.

The Stop Allergy Now Protocol includes a number of techniques that are each powerful and, in combination, can actually eliminate both symptoms and evidence of allergies in the blood. The techniques include:

- **NAET** (Nambudripad Allergy Elimination Technique), a procedure to correct the error in the brain by opening and aligning the body's energy pathways in the presence of the allergen so the brain no longer sees it as a threat.
- **NET** (Neuro-Emotional Technique) helps free us from unconstructive emotions that interfere with health and bodily function;
- **AK** (Applied Kinesiology) uses the body's muscle response to evaluate body function. It can trace irritation of the nervous system caused by mechanical, chemical, or emotional factors. (20)
- **TBM** (Total Body Modification) works on balancing the body's communication flow (physically, chemically, and emotionally) through the nervous

system; it ensures all communication lines are synchronized and working perfectly. Corrections might involve physical manipulation, nutritional changes, or direct energy correction.

- **Zone Healing** balances six physical zones in the body to improve the internal communication by recognizing and correcting unconstructive ideas and concepts.
- **25-Hour Dietary Change** desensitizes the body for specific allergens after each metabolic element and allergy treatment.
- **10-Day Detox Diet** preps the body for allergy elimination. Homeopathic supplements support body function during detox. This supports whatever allergy and emotion we want to clear in the allergy and elimination protocol process, or just to improve body function.
- **Nutritional and Herbal Supplements** support and correct the body during the allergy elimination protocol process.
- **Relaxation and Reprogramming** decrease stress that can negatively affect the immune system and improve the body's internal communication system.
- **Yoga Breathing** techniques exercise the nervous system and help it communicate with the digestive

system and cardiovascular system, so the body can handle oxygen correctly. (20)

I have studied additional techniques, like yoga, biofeedback, neuro-linguistic programming (NLP), hypnosis, and others, which have helped me create the Allergy Free Today Protocol to help patients actually eliminate allergy symptoms from their lives. This has been demonstrated by before-and-after blood results showing the complete elimination of symptoms for both physically identified and emotionally derived allergies.

Chapter 14: What Else Can I Do to Improve My Family's Health?

"A good laugh and a long sleep are the best cures in the doctor's book."

--Irish Proverb

In addition to the techniques we have talked about, there are some steps you can take by yourself to improve your health. These include physical activity, physical hygiene, good nutrition and hydration, emotional support, and proper sleep.

Physical Activity

Adding more walking to your day, not just in dedicated exercise, but in running errands and other daily activities will be beneficial to everyone. Walk to near places instead of driving. Park your car further away from your destination and walk. Take multiple short walks to break up your day. Five miles a day is a good goal.

To become even more fit, you can strengthen muscles with weights or resistance, training 20-40 minutes, three to four times a week. Stretch every joint for flexibility at least three to four times a week to keep the joints functioning. Practice some form of cardiovascular exercise, like 20-30 minutes of interval training, three to four times per week.

Good Hygiene

Make sure that you take a bath or shower every time you work up a sweat. If you play soccer, take a bike ride, or go to the gym, take a shower as soon as you get home. A little bit of hot water and soap does a great job of getting rid of the bugs and germs you collect from sweating and touching things that are dirty and germy, and then wiping your face.

Also, make it a strict rule to wash your hands before you eat or before you touch any of the holes in your face—eyes, mouth, ears, and nose. Wash your hands. Even if you just use water without soap. The most important thing is to have water running over them for at least 30 seconds. It is better if the water is on the warm side. It is even better if you use soap. Just instilling this habit before eating, you become healthier, because the germs that stress the immune system will have less opportunity to enter the body.

Research shows that most people who clean their hands with hand sanitizer all day actually stress the immune system by causing the natural bacteria-fighters to become lazy. The immune system is like the military. The soldiers need to practice all the time to prepare for a threat. If they were sitting around eating and drinking all day long, they would get fat and untrained. Then if there were an attack, they would not perform at their best. Having a little bit of stress, like ordinary bacteria that the immune system can easily get rid of, trains the immune system to be stronger and better. If we kill everything with external products and stay in a bubble, then when we open the bubble and expose ourselves to normal air, all the bugs will be strong, and the immune system will have no practice killing them, so it becomes overwhelmed.

Hand sanitizers can be useful when you do not have access to water, but do not make a habit of using them regularly. Use water as your primary cleaning measure, preferably with soap.

Eat for Wellness

Nutritional support gives the body what it needs: primarily fruits and vegetables to provide vitamins, minerals and fiber; protein to help us grow and develop; and oil to lubricate everything and provide nerve conduction and membranes for new cell growth. Starches are congestive for the body. The more we focus on pasta, bread, and processed foods–even homemade processed foods–the more congested the body and all its plumbing will be. The body will not function optimally.

You need to develop eating habits to support your body's normal functions that will be tasty, clean, and healthy. The most nutritious diet consists primarily of organic foods including vegetables, fruit, and protein (about the size of the palm of your hand) for each meal. The protein can be a combination of nuts, grain, meat, and fish.

Research shows that sugar stresses the immune system. If you have a soft drink with lunch, which contains about seven to nine teaspoons (15 grams) of sugar, your immune system will operate at 50% capacity for the next four to six hours. That means you are more vulnerable to all the germs and diseases floating around. If we add emotional stress—like someone criticizing you—we increase the chance that you will get sick, because your immune system is not strong enough to protect you. On top of that, if you originally had very severe, life-threatening allergies, even if we cleared them, they could flare up again. In a stressed immune system, the emotional memory can bring back symptoms, even if the blood is cleared.

Therefore, you want to make sure that you have as little processed sugar as possible in your diet. This does not include natural sugars in fruits, but refined sugar. Juices can also be very stressful. To make eight ounces of carrot juice, you need about 20 large carrots. Juices generally have a higher glycemic index than whole fruit, meaning they raise your blood sugar faster. Even something that seems less fruity, like carrot juice, can spike your blood sugar if you drink very much of it. Unlike an apple or orange, whose juice has only a slightly higher glycemic index, the glycemic index of carrots is very low, but carrot juice is almost double, putting it on par with high sugar fruit juices. If you drink eight ounces of fruit or carrot juice in the morning, you will get a lot of energy from the sugar, but your immune system will become very vulnerable. If you just drink a little bit, it is not a big deal, but eight ounces is too much. If it is daily, it can definitely stress the immune system. If you have fruit juice with every meal, it stresses the immune system for hours after every meal.

Aside from just avoiding sugar, you can use the elimination method discussed in Chapter 9 to determine what other foods cause reactions and avoid them.

Another thing that you can do to improve your health is cleaning from the inside. The detox program in the Allergy Free Today Protocol (see Resources) was designed to cleanse the body from the inside using a vegan diet for six to 21 days once to twice a year, so that food absorption, assimilation, and elimination improves. The body's communication systems improve and you function better overall.

If you have an issue with weight or emotional eating, train yourself to leave some food on your plate. This one step helps to put you in control of your eating. For more information, please refer to Daniel Amon's book, *The Daniel Plan: 40 Days to a Healthier Life* or Dr. Mark Hymon's book, *Eat Fat, Get Thin.*

Drinking Water

The amount of water we need to drink depends on our body weight. A good formula to use is that we should drink 50% of our weight in ounces. That means if you weigh 120 pounds, you should drink 60 ounces of water a day.

We should drink 16 to 24 ounces of water 15 minutes before each meal, not during the meal. Coffee is dehydrating, so if you drink coffee, you need to drink twice as much water for every cup of coffee.

Alcohol, juices and soda are not equivalent to water and do not count in your daily total.

Healthy Mind

Keeping a healthy mind is important to maintaining a healthy body. There are things you can stop doing as well as things you can start doing to improve your mental health.

The first step is to stop focusing on your fears, worries, and concerns. Choose a spot on your body that you designate as a delete button. Every time you find yourself thinking a negative thought, press on this spot and say, “Delete! Delete! Delete!” Then focus on what you want in a positive way.

For example, if you are thinking about not having enough money, press your delete button and say aloud, “Delete! Delete! Delete!” Then change your thoughts to the money you would like to have flowing to you and how good this will feel. Be careful that you frame your new thoughts in the positive, such as “I look forward to more money coming my way,” rather than a negative thought like “I look forward to not being broke.” The latter is still focusing on your broke-ness. The third step is to ask yourself, “What action should I take to achieve what I want?” Start taking the actions that you come up with.

Another great way to improve your mental and physical health is meditation. Today you do not need 20 years to learn to meditate well. You can take a shortcut by listening to the right music to put you into a meditative state. Holosync by Bill Harris is a great meditation series to clear your emotional state, balance and synchronize your brain, and increase relaxation.

Laughter really is the best medicine. One of the simplest and easiest ways to improve your state of mind is to laugh. If you do not have anything else handy to laugh about, you can do this laughter exercise: Every hour, look up at the ceiling and laugh out loud for 30 to 60 seconds. In two to three days, you will feel like a happier and more positive person. This will improve your immune system. The average child laughs 200 to 300 times per day. The average adult laughs only seven times a day. Increase your laughter, improve your health.

Emotional Support for Your Family

Emotional support is very important. Research shows that if you constantly tell your child she is stupid, she will start to perform poorly and do stupid things. If you tell her she is smart, she will start to perform well and be smart. In one study, researchers told teachers that their classes of average students were high performers. Because the teachers expected the students to do better than average, they did perform better than average. (The way you talk to yourself can have an equally profound effect.)

It is important to understand what stressors at home, at school, or in the world affect you or your child, so you can develop coping strategies and prevent stress from weakening the immune system.

For example, one day your child does not want to go to school. You can just force your child to go to school without any discussion, or you can investigate why your child does not want to go. The better you understand your child, the easier it is to start ruling out possibilities, since they usually will not volunteer the reason. A conversation might go like this:

Child: "I don't want to go to school."

Parent: "Why don't you want to go to school?"

Child: "I don't like school."

Parent: "What don't you like about school?"

Child: "I don't know."

Parent: "Do you have a problem with kids who sit near you in class?"

Child: "No."

Parent: "Is it a problem with the teacher? Did she say something to you to hurt your feelings?"

Child: "No."

Parent: "Is this about lunch?"

Child: Silence.

Parent: "Did your friend not want to sit with you yesterday? Is that what happened?"

Child: "Yes! I had to eat lunch alone and I don't like to sit by myself at lunch. She left me to go sit with someone else and she didn't want to sit with me."

Now that we have found the problem, we need to find a solution. You could say, "Maybe you could sit with somebody else who is sitting alone. How do you think that other person sitting alone feels?"

Offer some simple ideas and let your child come up with ideas on her own – sit with another person, try to see if you can join the table where your friend is sitting, etc. First let the child handle the situation.

I will relate a story from my personal experience. My son came to me and said he did not want to go to his karate training. When I asked why, he said it was because he just had a haircut and it was too short, and everyone was going to make fun of him. I asked who was going to make fun of him, and he told me the name of the boy he thought was going to make fun of him. I said, "You know what? I am going to come with you to class, and wait until this other boy arrives. If he says anything about your haircut, I will confront him about it. But if he doesn't say anything, we can just let it go."

He agreed and went to class. I waited to see if the other boy showed up to class, and he did. My son was just waiting for the other boy to laugh at him and make fun of his haircut. However, it just so happened that the other boy had also gotten a haircut and was feeling self-conscious about his own hair. He did not even care about my son's haircut because he was busy worrying about his own.

When the class was over, I asked my son if anything happened and he said no, the other boy just criticized his own haircut and talked about how mad he was that his parents forced him to make it shorter. The situation my son wanted to avoid did not even occur. However, if we hadn't come up with a coping strategy, my son would have missed his class out of fear of something that never happened.

It is our job as parents to get involved in our kids' lives, to listen to them, and try to help them find solutions for themselves. If they fail, then get involved. Providing this emotional support helps kids become stronger because when kids feel good about themselves and their ability to cope, their immune systems become stronger.

Even as adults, we start with something insignificant and blow it completely out of proportion in our minds. The feelings we have about the bad things we imagine could happen, stop us from moving forward. However, the feelings are real, and they are causing stress in the body, so it is important to address them.

When we are feeling depressed, unhappy or anxious, the immune system slowly starts to shut down, reducing our protection and making us more susceptible to illness.

We want to make sure our immune system is functioning fully at all times. If we have done all the work to strengthen the metabolic system and remove the allergies, we want to keep a balanced emotional state to take it to the next level of ironclad protection.

Sleep Yourself Well

Getting enough sleep is highly correlated with improved mental and physical health. Your body needs four to five hours of deep sleep every night. Most people need seven to nine hours of sleep to get four to five hours of deep sleep. A few people – some yogis, for example – manage to get more deep sleep in a shorter time and stay rested and in good health. Eighty-five percent of all healing and recovery happens in your sleep.

Your Health Care Partner

To improve your overall health, it is important to find a doctor who can work with you to help improve the body's health functions – integrative doctors, applied kinesiology doctors, or other doctors that use the techniques previously mentioned in this book. There are also many kinds of general support you can give your family and yourself to maintain optimal health.

Chapter 15: Success Stories

"It always seems impossible until it's done."
--Nelson Mandela

Cheryl-Osteoporosis

Cheryl's case was the first time I investigated the role of allergies with seemingly unrelated symptoms. Cheryl, who was in her late thirties, came to me with a lot of pain in her back. She said she was bending forward to pick up a bottle of water when she threw her back out. She could not stand up. She was sitting there until her boyfriend helped her up and brought her to the office. She exercised four or five times a week. She was doing stretching, resistance, and running. I did not understand why bending forward to pick up an empty bottle would create this pain.

I sent her to get X-rays, which showed that she already had greater than 50% osteoporosis. I did not understand how a person of this age who was active, exercised, and ate well could have over 50% osteoporosis. We sent her for a bone density test, which confirmed close to 60% bone loss. I started checking with all my colleagues and doctor friends to see what I could do for her. One of them said, maybe she is allergic to calcium. I did not understand how a person could be allergic to calcium, because this is an essential element of the body. However, I followed his guidance, I learned the method, and I treated her calcium sensitivity. I sent her back six months later to repeat the bone density analysis. The second bone density test showed no osteoporosis.

The company who ran the test said that they must have made a mistake the first time, because they had never seen anyone go from 60% bone loss to no bone loss without medication. They thought there must be something wrong with their machine. I told them that I had treated her for calcium sensitivity, and this was the result I was looking for. We took another X-ray and it showed no sign of osteoporosis.

This happened in 1995 and it inspired me to learn more about this technique and to learn how it could help more and more people.

Eva—Kidney function and emotional transformation

When Eva came to me, she was in her 20s. She had been on dialysis for kidney problems for four years and had lupus. She consulted me for a second opinion to see if I could do anything to improve her kidneys before they removed them from her body. She had been a professional dancer and could not dance any more. She was on 100% disability. She was connected to a dialysis machine, which in those days went through her stomach, lying on her back for 12 hours every day. This was her protocol when I met her.

She was allergic to many different things that we cleared slowly one by one. Then we worked on the kidneys. We gave her tonifying herbs and nutritional supplements to make her stronger. Although we treated the kidneys for a long time to make the kidneys stronger, they did not stay strong.

I decided we needed to work more on her emotions. When we reviewed her life history to find the root cause of her condition, we learned that she had a lot of fear. Both Eva's father and mother abused her. As a child, her father kidnapped her three times. Her criminal father kept her in hiding. When her father went to jail, she went back to her mother and Eva continued to live with a lot of negative emotions and fear. Every night when she went to sleep, she did not know whether she would wake up in the morning in the same place.

When I dug deeper into her fear, she told me a story about being kidnapped and staying with her father who let her watch *The Wizard of Oz* every night. She was so scared of the green witch that every night for years when she went to sleep, she was afraid that the green witch would come and hurt her or kill her.

We worked on treatments to release many emotions. *The Wizard of Oz* still really seemed to hold her emotions hostage. I asked her, "Do you remember how the witch dies?" "Yes, a bucket of water," she said.

I suggested that she try putting a glass of water by her bed every night before going to sleep, so that if the wicked witch came, she could throw the water on her. This was enough to stop the wicked witch from ever appearing in her dreams again because she had a logical solution to the witch.

In six months, she completely healed. As of the printing of this book, this is the only case in the United States where the kidneys healed completely with normal function after four years of continuous support on a dialysis machine. At the beginning, they reduced dialysis time to eight hours, then four hours, then four hours every other day, then once a week. Then they decided that her kidneys had begun to function well enough to function perfectly on their own.

Although I never directly treated the lupus, I just made her body stronger and stronger, physically, emotionally, and energetically. When we tested her blood to check for lupus, there was no longer any sign of it in her blood. She stopped coming to my office. I met her again five years later and there was still no sign of kidney problems or lupus. Her diseases completely disappeared after we improved her metabolic function supporting her organs, eliminated her allergies, and eliminated her fears.

Lucien-Anaphylactic reaction to peanuts

Lucien's mother brought him to me when he was less than two years old. He was allergic to peanuts, walnuts, shrimp, and white rice—all at the anaphylactic level. His mother needed to use an EpiPen injection twice to save his life before coming to see me. He also had a skin disorder that did not respond to any treatment, so the pediatrician referred them to me. In a few months, the skin condition completely healed after I corrected his metabolic function. In addition to the severe allergies listed above, he had allergies to many environmental and food factors including trees, pollen, flowers, weeds, grass, dogs, and cats. We cleared everything.

When we did the pre-treatment blood analysis, the results showed peanuts and walnuts as Class 4, which is anaphylactic. We did the test again one year later when we finished the entire protocol, and walnuts was reduced from Class 4 to zero, and peanuts from four to Class 1. Then, with a medical doctor supervising, we exposed him to walnuts and peanuts, actually eating them, and he had no symptoms, no reaction. He said he does not like the taste of peanuts, and that is perfectly okay. The important thing is he is no longer allergic to them.

In addition to the basic blood test for peanut allergy, another test can measure reactions to each of the seven peanut protein molecules. At first testing, this test showed that he was allergic to six of the seven proteins. When we repeated the test after treatment, he was allergic to only one of the seven proteins. We still wanted to clear that residual allergy permanently, so we continued treatment. We succeeded in eliminating the reaction to that last peanut protein molecule and lowering the peanut's class from one to zero.

Darius-Allergic to everything

Darius was five years old when his mother brought him to me. His waist was 36 inches and he weighed 100 pounds. His blood test revealed that he was allergic to 65 different things. He was allergic to the entire menu of everything they ate at home and everything around the house, from grass to dogs to trees. We worked with him for a little over a year and cleared 62 allergies. We reduced the remaining three allergies, but we could not clear them 100%. Eventually, over time, his body returned to normal weight. He moved away before we were able to clear the last three allergies. He remained allergic to wheat, corn, and dairy. Now Darius has grown up and has a son of his own. His son inherited these three allergies, but none of the other 62. Therefore, it is interesting to see that this technique actually eliminated these allergies from the next generation. Today we have additional tools that would have helped clear the final three.

Matthew-Autism

Matthew, a seven-year-old autistic boy, came to me with many behavioral issues. He could not read or write. He was screaming (almost like Turret's), cursing, yelling, and not really participating. They lived far away, so they could only come for allergy elimination treatment once a week. It was a big commitment by the father, who stopped working to take care of his son.

A year later, Matthew would run to give me a hug and kiss when he got to the office. He talked; he learned reading and writing, and he began participating. This was a dramatic improvement.

Raya-Psoriasis and painful eczema

Raya came to me with very painful eczema and psoriasis, which she had had for over ten years. It started later in life; she was not born with it. She said she did not believe in what I do because it was not medicine. Her father was a medical doctor and her mother was a psychiatrist. However, she was willing to try because she had already tried everything medical doctors could offer and none of the medications helped. I worked with her for four months and the psoriasis and eczema completely disappeared, and she had no more pain.

Raya had another unusual symptom: a white, powder-like substance coated the skin over her chest. She also sometimes had puss coming from her skin. All of that completely disappeared. After four months, before we even finished the entire protocol, all the symptoms were gone.

Reza-Pollen and dust allergy

Reza moved to Los Angeles many years ago. Every spring and summer, his allergies to pollen and dust flared up. He became congested, could not breathe, and required many antihistamines. After we cleared the pollen and dust allergies, it was the first spring and summer since Reza moved to LA that he did not have to use medication even once.

During the second year, we had strong Santa Ana winds and he reacted to that. He knew from our training how to collect a sample of the air that was blowing in and brought it in to clear it. We were able to clear the exact allergens that were causing the problem, even though he did not know exactly what was in the sample.

Justin-Asthma problem

Justin came to me as an eight-year-old with serious asthma. He had three different inhalers that he used three to four times a day. I wanted to see what level of distress Justin reached before he used his inhaler, so I asked him to rate his need for the inhaler each time he reached for it on a scale of one to ten, with one being just a little bit, and 10 being that he feels like he's going to die. He said it was usually between five and eight. It really affected him emotionally.

We started clearing the allergies, and by the time we cleared all the basic allergies, he started to feel better, stopped using the daily inhaler and only used the one he used at night. A few months later, he stopped using all of them and could function very well.

PE class did not stress him out any more and he went from being an anxious kid on the sidelines to being a fun-loving participant. I reduced his treatments to once a month for maintenance. Six months later, after he was completely cleared, he got a sick and used the inhaler, but it was the only time he used it in months.

I never did any specific treatment for asthma with him. We just cleared the biomechanical functions, the metabolic functions and the things he was allergic to, and his body was able to do the rest.

Lisa—Concentration and focusing

Nine-year-old Lisa had trouble with concentration, almost to the extent of ADD. She was very talented and creative. She loved drawing, but could not focus. It got to the point where they had to move her to a different school because she was doing very poorly in class.

They lived in the Valley in Los Angeles, so they came only when they could—sometimes after school, sometimes on the weekend. When we cleared the allergies, her performance improved so dramatically that she started acing every single class and she became the best soccer player in the school. She was chosen to represent the school in a girl's soccer competition. She is quick and knows how to control the ball.

I did something differently with her. I found that when she was not able to express her artistic side, it created a lot of frustration and was holding her back. I asked her parents to give her permission when she feels stressed to express her frustration on paper. So they let her draw whenever she was stressed. This difference contributed to her healing.

Nancy—Watery eyes

Nancy was a young woman in her mid-20s who was using multiple allergy medications including inhalers. One of the things that affected her dramatically was her eyes. Her eyes watered so badly that it impaired her vision when she was driving to work.

When we cleared the basic metabolic panel, most of the symptoms disappeared and she was able to reduce her medication use by 75%. When we did the blood analysis, we found that most of her allergies were environmental. When we cleared the environmental panel, all the symptoms disappeared completely. She was very happy not to have any more symptoms and was not concerned about having another blood test right away, but we did repeat the blood test about a year later and it showed no more allergies.

Barbara–Hay fever

Barbara was a teacher in her late 30s. She was taking medications for severe nasal allergy symptoms, like runny nose and sneezing. She needed to eliminate these symptoms to function better at work and at home. When we finished the metabolic panel, all of the symptoms disappeared, so we did not actually need to treat any environmental or food allergies. Because we balanced her metabolic function, it allowed her immune system to stop producing allergy symptoms. She was able to stop her allergy medication, which caused withdrawal headaches for a couple days, but from one visit to the next, the headaches went away.

Jeremy-Severe sinus issues

Jeremy came to Los Angeles from Texas in his early 30s to become an actor. He had major sinus issues, including frequent nosebleeds. His medical doctor recommended surgery to open up his sinuses, but he did not want to do surgery, so he came to me. He started to feel better after the metabolic panel. Then we did the blood test and treated the rest of his allergies over time between his filming schedules. It took longer because he had to take breaks for several months at a time for filming. Then we would work intensively during his breaks. After we cleared environmental and food allergies, his symptoms stopped, and his blood test showed his allergies completely cleared.

Testimonials

"I could sing the praises of Dr. Orpelli for many pages, however, that wouldn't be appropriate here. What needs to be said in brief is that I suffered consistently for almost 10 years with painful eczema over much of my body. I was fortunate to meet Dr. Orpelli and, within three months of regular treatments, I was relieved of most of my discomfort, as well as able to stop taking very strong antihistamines throughout the day. This remains to be the case four months later. If you suspect your system is out of balance, or you have diagnosed allergies, I would strongly urge you to consult Dr. Orpelli, learn about Stop Allergy Now, and take advantage of his knowledge and dedication to helping his patients." **--Joan Durham**

"When my daughter was about three months old she had baby acne that wasn't going away, Dr. Orpelli cleared her acne in one visit! Later she developed eczema, which she got from my genes, and through the Stop Allergy Now process her eczema is gone!" **--Kalaya Bhaedhyajibh**

"My son went to Dr. Orpelli because of his eczema and anaphylactic reaction to peanuts, walnuts, shrimp, and rice. The eczema was all over his body. After only one month his skin improved to 80% after one year all of his allergies are gone and the blood results showed no allergies. Dr. Orpelli was very patient and sensitive to us. He is really good with children and knows how to get their trust so that he can work with them. He explained everything very clearly and sometimes even twice, since English is not my first language. He is very kind, knowledgeable, and has good sense of humor. We enjoyed working with him and I am looking forward to visiting him to clear my allergies, too."

--Doreen Desse

“In order to help people understand what Dr. Orpelli can do, and Stop Allergy Now, I wanted to provide some details on my experience. While it’s best to just talk to Dr. Orpelli, as he's so down to earth, knowledgeable, and easy to talk to, it can sometimes help to hear the experience of a patient as well.

When our family pediatrician mentioned Stop Allergy Now to eliminate allergies, as practiced by Dr. Orpelli, I was very curious, as our children have suffered strong allergy symptoms since birth. Our pediatrician is great at exploring a variety of options to best help his patients, and has really been focused on finding help for allergies. I trust the thorough due diligence process he conducts before making any recommendations or referrals.

The Stop Allergy Now treatment includes using kinesiology to identify allergens and acupuncture with pressure points, not needles, to clear the body of the allergy. It can be hard to wrap your head around it, but the results speak for themselves. My one-year-old daughter has been severely allergic to breast milk as well as a few other foods, and has always had a very low appetite and constipation issues. I've tried many routes to both identify the source of her issues and to try treat her symptoms.

At the appointment with Dr. Orpelli, he started with a chiropractic adjustment using a high tech clicker machine on an area of the spine around the neck, which is directly tied to the digestive system, since I talked about her severe constipation. Then he did the Stop Allergy Now treatment, in which he uses a laser light for the acupuncture points on kids. This is TMI, but such an important result to share, as after that treatment, she pooped three times in 12 hours, after not pooping for five days. In fact, every time we go to Dr. Orpelli, her digestive system seems to have an immediate positive reaction. She is now eating much better and much more regular. I can also tell that certain foods, such as dairy products, which he's identified as an allergy and cleared from the body with Stop Allergy Now treatment, no longer have the negative effect on her as they did before.

I can’t imagine what people go through in life with severe allergies that trigger anaphylactic shock and the constant worry and carrying around an EpiPen. While I cannot attest to the treatment of allergies of this severity, Dr. Orpelli has some great patient stories to share! It just makes sense to give Stop Allergy Now a try if it has the possibility of literally clearing the body's reaction. Plus, once the allergy is cleared, it's cleared for good. It seems so crazy, but it is really cool to learn and watch it work."

--Shannon Carlson

"Highly recommended. Genius doctor! I was very sick for two months. There were no doctors who were helping, each doctor's recommendation made my condition worse. A colleague suggested Dr. Orpelli, as she had worked with him to great success. I showed up very skeptical. I am still in the midst of treatments. Within one week Dr. Orpelli cleared up my symptoms. He then started to build up my body and tolerance by fixing my metabolic function and remove my symptoms. We are continuing to work together as I get healthier and healthier. He's the only one who knew what was wrong in my body and how to correct it. I am deeply grateful and indebted. Follow what he says and you will get better. Highly recommended. A+" **--Debbi Johnson**

"Recently I started working with Dr. Orpelli to eliminate my allergy. It is very helpful; I no longer need a daily antihistamine. The Stop Allergy Now process requires discipline and is no magic cure, but it is worth the time. It really works."

--Michael Rosen

"Dr Orpelli not only eliminated pain in my neck, shoulder, and hip, he recently reduced my allergy symptoms after two treatments.

In addition, his constant research on health and science resulted in early awareness of nutritional supplements, years before they became common. I feel confident in his care and greatly appreciate how he shares his well-researched health maintenance supplements and exercises with patients."**--Karen Hernandez**

"I would just like to say that Dr. Aaron Orpelli is one of the most compassionate and truly gifted doctors I've ever been to. He truly cares about his patients in a way we always wish from doctors, but rarely see. Dr. Orpelli goes beyond the call of duty, time and time again. He is always seeking new and innovative ways to bring his patients to complete wellness and health. Where other doctors have dismissed my case as too complicated or incurable, Dr. Orpelli has never given up on me. It is thanks to him and the many techniques and treatments he practices that I'm even walking today." **--Juliana Zanville**

"I had many nagging problems like allergies and eczema, which my Western medical doctors could not fix. Dr. O. has a lot of tricks up his sleeve that helped me. My Stop Allergy Now protocol included NAET, NET, Zone Healing, Kinesiology, chiropractic, acupuncture, nutrition, relaxation, and diet. My issues have been virtually eliminated. **--Dov Kelemer**

"I came to Dr. Orpelli with a problem it seemed like no Western doctor could understand or fix. There was no cure but time. His knowledge of flushing out toxins and cleaning the body changed me within days of beginning his prescribed protocol. After several months of his treatment, I felt stronger and healthier. He is an excellent coach and cheerleader for wellness."

--Sarah Jo Marks

"A must read book for any one suffering from allergies. In this groundbreaking, simple-to-read and follow book, Dr. Orpelli explains how you can take charge of your allergies today and live an allergy-free,healthy life. Application of knowledge from his material will change your world of health for the better."

--Bala G. Gopurala M.Sc.,M.D.

American Board of Internal Medicine
Board Certified Medical Oncologist and
an Integrative Medicine Practitioner

"Dr. Orpelli has tried to inform readers through his book, Allergy Free Today, about possible encounters with known and hidden allergies in their daily lives. This book is very informative for patients from all walks of life. I congratulate Dr. Orpelli for his enthusiasm and willingness to share this valuable information with the readers who are desperately searching for a way out of the clutches of allergies and trying to live a normal life. I highly recommend this book for anyone who truly wants to be set free from allergies and sensitivities of all kinds."

--Devi S. Nambudripad
M.D., D.C., L.Ac., Ph.D.

Resources

"I am still learning."
--Michelangelo

Please visit http://www.AllergyFreeToday.com/gift to download:

1. A list of allergy-safe foods.
2. A diagram showing the location of the rib point to check to see if you have been exposed to an allergen.
3. Detox Diet

Recommended Reading

The Daniel Plan: 40 Days to a Healthier Life by Daniel Amon

Eat Fat, Get Thin by Dr. Mark Hymon

The Food Solution by Cari Schaefer M.A., TCM, L.Ac.

Thresholds of the Mind by Bill Harris

Bibliography

1. **Prevention, Centers for Disease Control and.** Health Data Interactive. *National Center for Health Statistics.* [Online] Centers for Disease Control and Prevention, 2012-2014. [Cited: May 16, 2016.] <http://www.cdc.gov/nchs/hdi/index.htm>.

2. **Diseases, National Institute of Allergy and Infectious.** National Institute of Allergy and Infectious Diseases. *National Institutes of Health, U.S. Department of Health and Human Services.* [Online] July 2012. <https://www.niaid.nih.gov/topics/foodAllergy/Documents/foodallergy.pdf.>

3. **Simons, F Estelle.** *Ancestors of Allergy.* New York: Global Medical Communications, 1994.

4. **Moses Maimonides, Suessman Muntner (editor).** *Treatise on Asthma (the Medical Writings of Moses Maimonides).* s.l. : J. B. Lippencott Company, 1963.

5. Antihistamine. *Medical discoveries.* [Online] [Cited: June 6, 2016.] <http://www.discoveriesinmedicine.com/A-An/Antihistamine.html>.

6. **Chavez, Donna M.** Theron Randolph, M.D.: An example for us all. *Natural world Healing.* [Online] 2001. [Cited: June 6, 2016.] <http://www.naturalworldhealing.com/allergy-randolph-champion.htm>.

7. **Sullivan, Ronald.** Theron G. Randolph, 89, Environmental Allergist. *The New York Times.* [Online] October 5, 1995. [Cited: June 6, 2016.] <http://www.nytimes.com/1995/10/05/us/theron-g-randolph-89-environmental-allergist.html>.

8. Dr. George Goodheart. *International College of Applied Kinesiology USA.* [Online] [Cited: June 6, 2016.] <http://www.icakusa.com/content/dr-george-goodheart>.

9. George Goodheart. *Wikipedia.* [Online] May 30, 2016. [Cited: June 6, 2016.] <https://en.wikipedia.org/wiki/George_Goodheart>.

10. **Horowitz, Janice M.** The Man with the Magic Fingers. *Time.* [Online] April 23, 2001. [Cited: June 6, 2016.] <http://content.time.com/time/magazine/article/0,9171,1956520,00.html>.

11. **Arthur F. Coca, M.D.** *The Pulse Test.* New york : Lyle Stuart, 1956.

12. **Gerasimo, Pilar.** Emotional Biochemistry. *Experience Life.* [Online] December 2003. [Cited: June 10, 2016.] <https://experiencelife.com/article/emotional-biochemistry/>.

13. *New findings of the correlation between acupoints and corresponding brain cortices using functional MRI.* **Z. H. Cho, S. C. Chung, J. P. Jones, J. B. Park, et al.** s.l.: The National Academy of Sciences, 1997.

14. **Krebs, Dr. Charles T.** Acupressure Effects on Brain Function. *Integrated Learning Enhancement Acupressure Program.* [Online] [Cited: June 10, 2016.] <http://i-leap.org/pdfs/Acupressure_Affects_on_Brain_-_150508_.pdf>.

15. **Education, Discovery.** Human Body: Pushing the Limits - Sensation - Teachers Guide. *Discovery Education.* [Online] 2008. [Cited: June 6, 2016.] <http://store.discoveryeducation.com/images/sites/42/pdf/DC023301TG.pdf>.

16. **NeuroBill.** How much data does the human brain process per second? *Reddit.* [Online] March 3, 2015. <https://www.reddit.com/r/askscience/comments/2xtz6n/how_much_data_does_the_human_brain_process_per/>.

17. **Markowsky, George.** Information Theory: Mathematics: Physiology. *Encyclopaedia Brittanica.* [Online] June 8, 2015. [Cited: June 6, 2016.] <http://www.britannica.com/topic/information-theory/Physiology>.

18. **Moss, Michael.** The Extraordinary Science of Addictive Junk Food. *The New York Times Magazine.* [Online] February 20, 2013. [Cited: June 6, 2016.]

<http://www.nytimes.com/2013/02/24/magazine/the-extraordinary-science-of-junk-food.html>.

19. **News, ABC.** Could Oreos Be as Addictive as Cocaine? . *ABC News.* [Online] October 16, 2013. [Cited: June 6, 2016.] <http://abcnews.go.com/Health/oreos-addictive-cocaine/story?id=20590182>.

20. *Digestive Mastery - Nutritional Protocols.* **Walter H. Schmidt, DC, DIBAK, DABCN.** 2014.

21. Sun Safety. *American Skin Association.* [Online] [Cited: June 6, 2016.] <http://www.americanskin.org/resource/safety.php>.

22. Sunburn. *WebMD.* [Online] April 11, 2014. [Cited: June 6, 2016.] <http://www.webmd.com/skin-problems-and-treatments/guide/sunburn?page>.

23. **Paige Bierma, M.A.** The Immune System and Stress. *Healthy Day.* [Online] January 20, 2016. <https://consumer.healthday.com/encyclopedia/stress-management-37/stress-health-news-640/the-immune-system-and-stress-645924.html>.

24. *Trauma equals danger—damage control by the immune system.* **Veit M. Stoecklein, Akinori Osuka, and James A. Lederer.** 2012, Journal of Leukocyte Biology, pp. 539-551.

25. *Psychological Stress and the Human Immune System: A Meta-Analytic Study of 30 Years of Inquiry.* **Segerstrom, Suzanne C. and Miller, Gregory E.** 4, s.l.: Psychological Bulletin, 2004, Vol. 130.

26. Brain Basics: Understanding Sleep. *National Institute of Neurological Disorders and Stroke.* [Online] National Institutes of Health, July 25, 2014. [Cited: May 15, 2016.] <http://www.ninds.nih.gov/disorders/brain_basics/understanding_sleep.htm>.

Made in the USA
Monee, IL
04 November 2026

67384889R00059